Dedicated to all of the two-minute brushers...

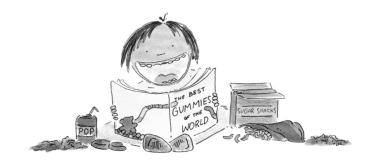

Published by Mrs. Weisz Books, Chicago, IL, USA

SUGAR BUGS

Sugar Bugs/written by Dr. Sam Weisz and Erica Weisz; illustrated by Erica Weisz. - 1st ed.

ISBN 978-0-9888338-1-4

1.Dentist - Juvenile Literature 2.Oral Hygiene - Juvenile Literature 3.Teeth - Juvenile Literature. I.Title.
The artwork was created in ink with watercolor and mixed media.
Book design by Erica Weisz

First Edition: 2014
10 9 8 7 6 5 4 3 2 1
www.mrsweiszbooks.com

SUGAR BUGS

Dr. Sam Weisz

Erica Weisz

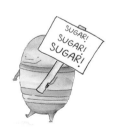

Life was easy for the Mutans family since they moved into the mouth of a young boy named Robbie.

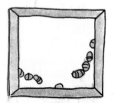 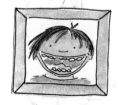 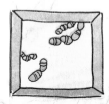

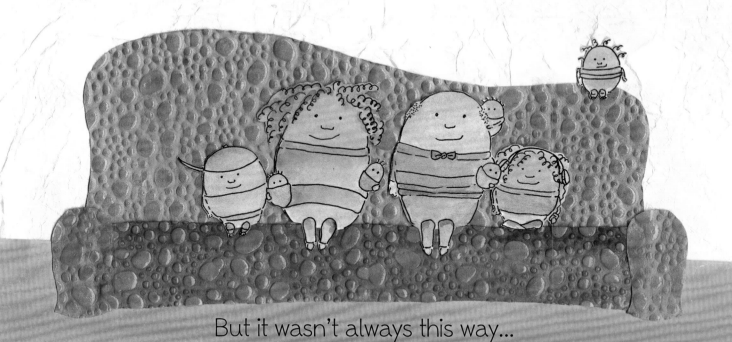

But it wasn't always this way...

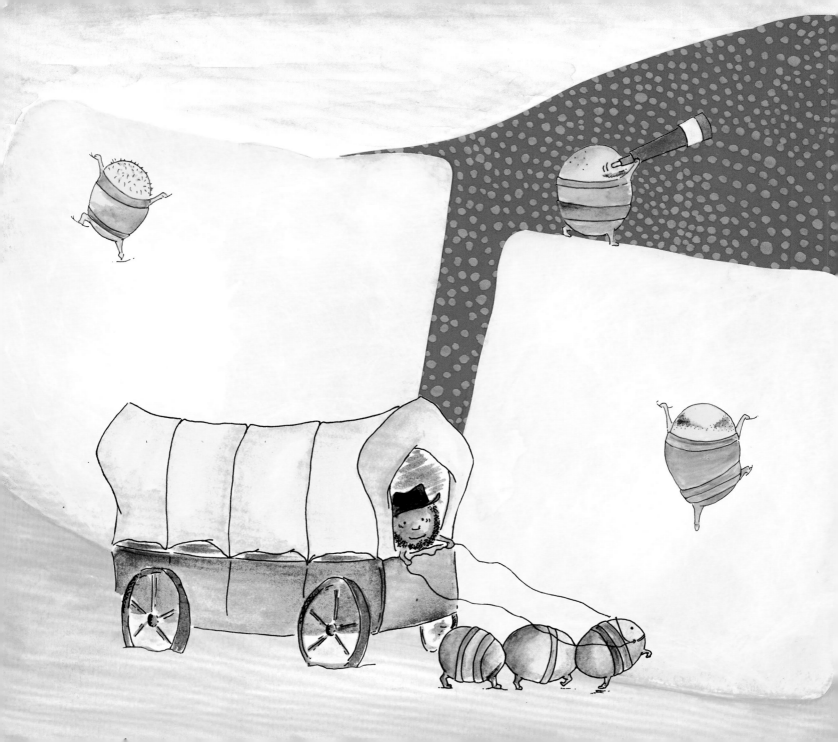

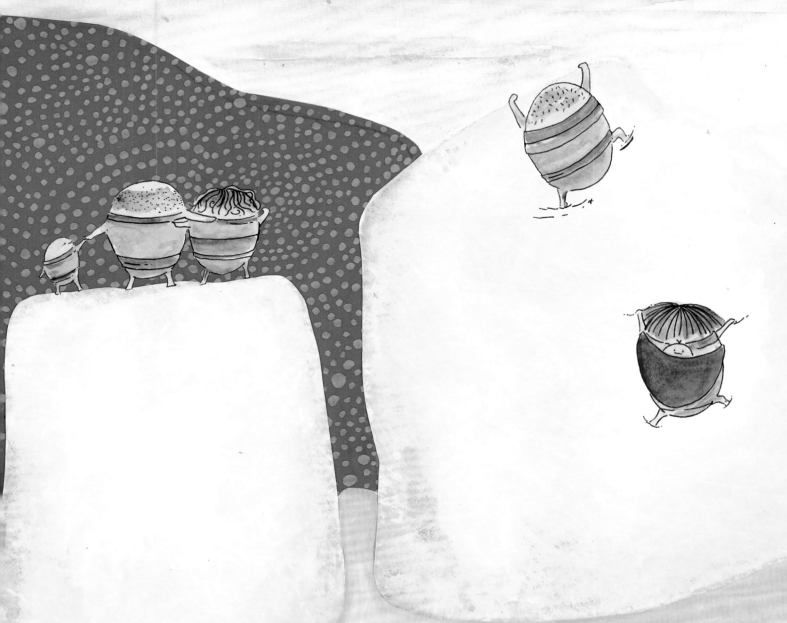

The Mutans family were some of the first sugar bug explorers.

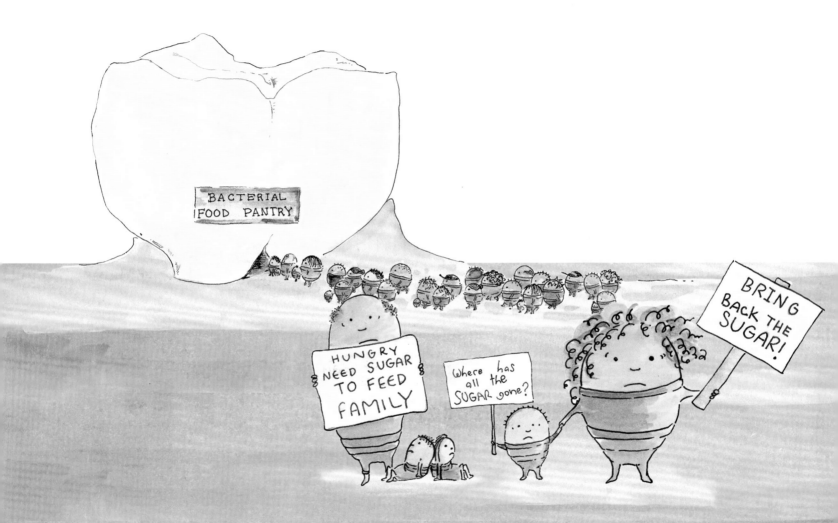

It was a hard life for all sugar bugs. A messy mouth filled with sticky, gooey sweets was not easy to find.

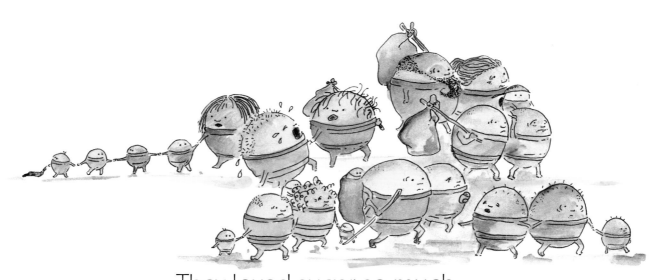

They loved sugar so much.
When it became scarce, all the sugar bugs were forced
to leave their mouth homes behind.

Finally, the Mutans found Robbie's mouth.

They fell in love!

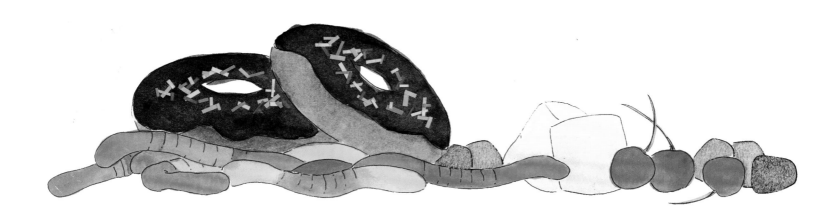

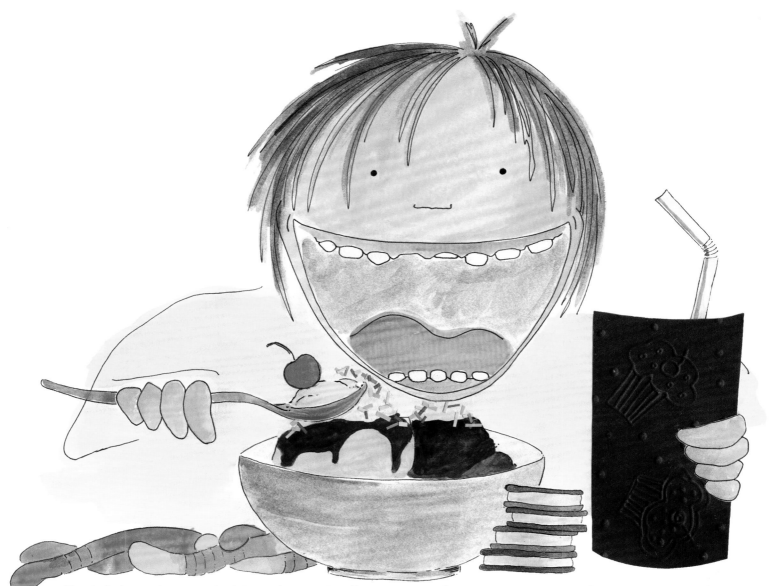

Robbie ate sprinkle donuts for breakfast, lollipops for lunch, and gummies for dinner. He took great care of the Mutans.

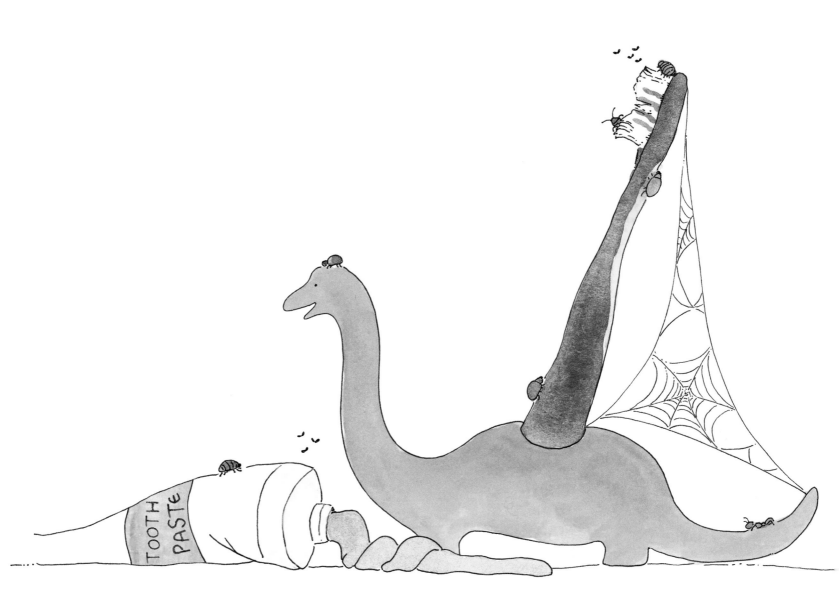

His toothbrush sat on the bathroom floor for days.

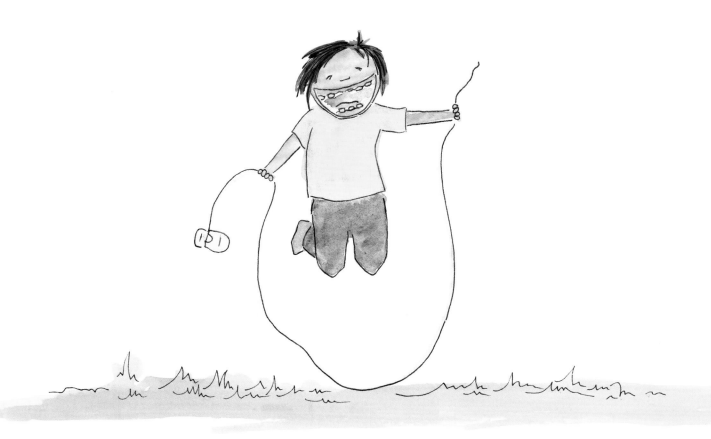

Robbie only used his floss for jump rope.

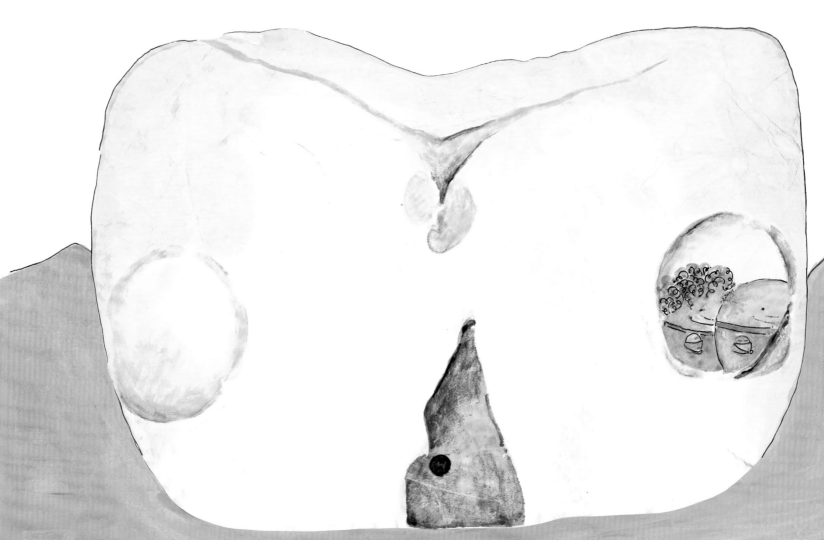

His molar tooth became the Mutans' new home
with a silky pink yard of gums.

The sugar bug children enjoyed playing for hours
in the open park where Robbie's baby tooth had been.

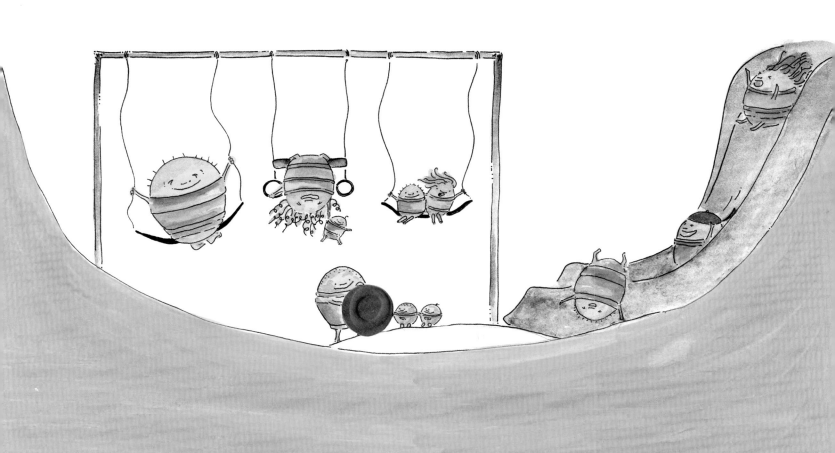

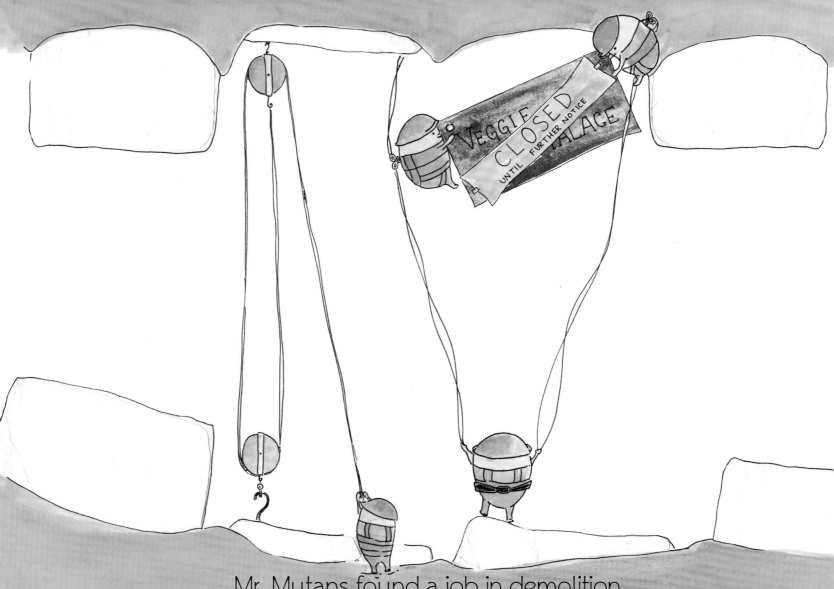

Mr. Mutans found a job in demolition,
tearing down homes and restaurants.

Mrs. Mutans was a stay-at-home mom,
teaching her children the tricks of being nasty little sugar bugs.

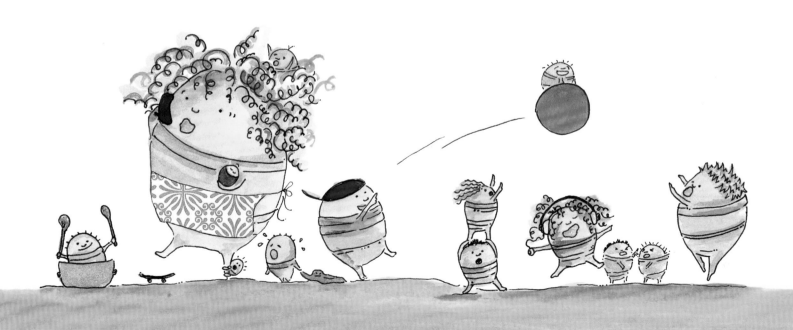

Life was perfect!

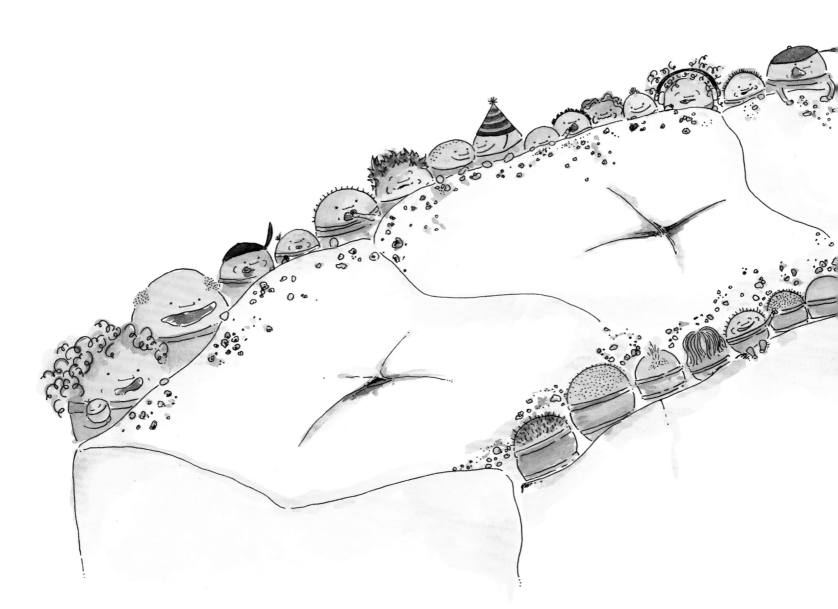

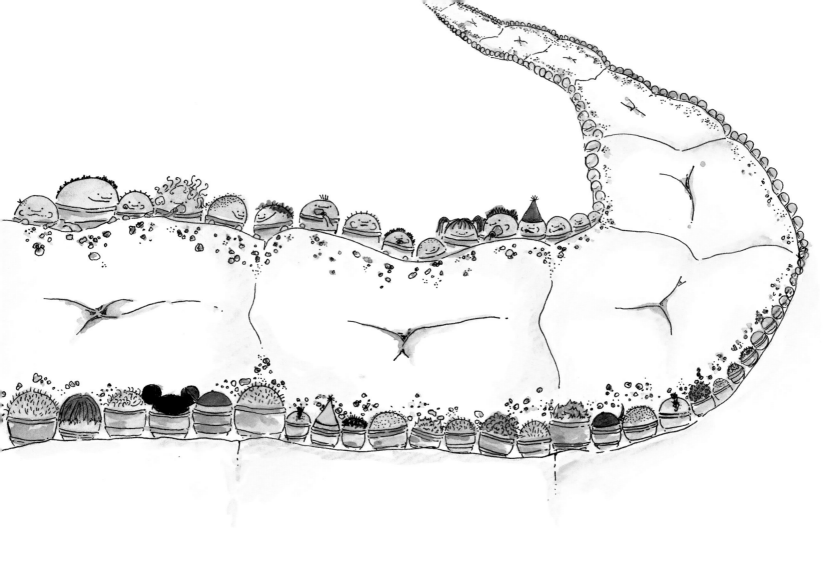

As their family multiplied by the day, the Mutans ate more
and more of the sweets never brushed away by Robbie.

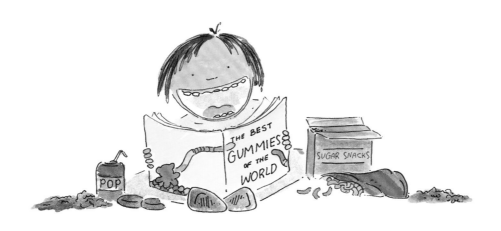

Over the next few months, the Mutans family
lived happily without Robbie knowing.

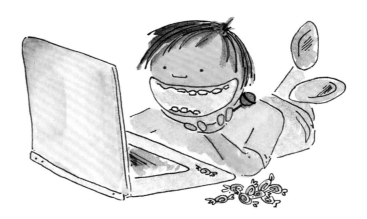

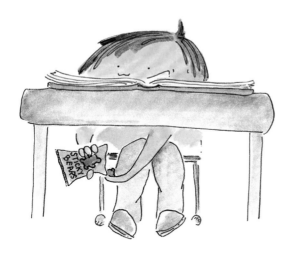

But then things started to change...

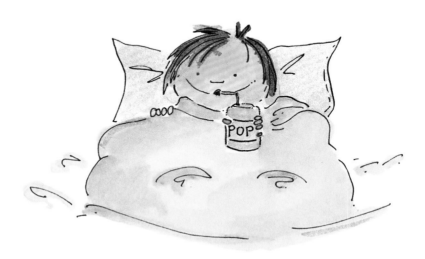

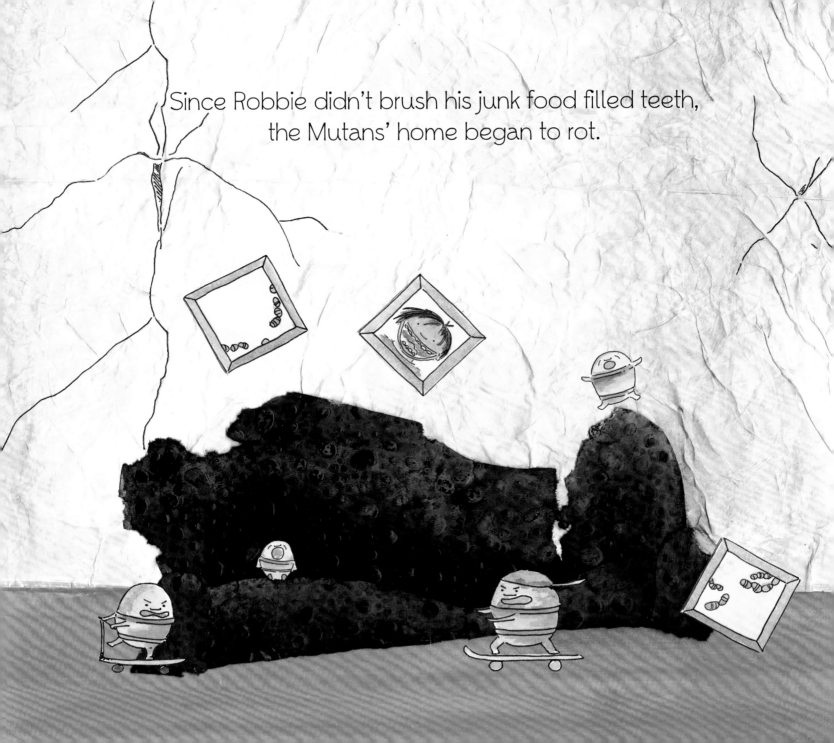

Since Robbie didn't brush his junk food filled teeth,
the Mutans' home began to rot.

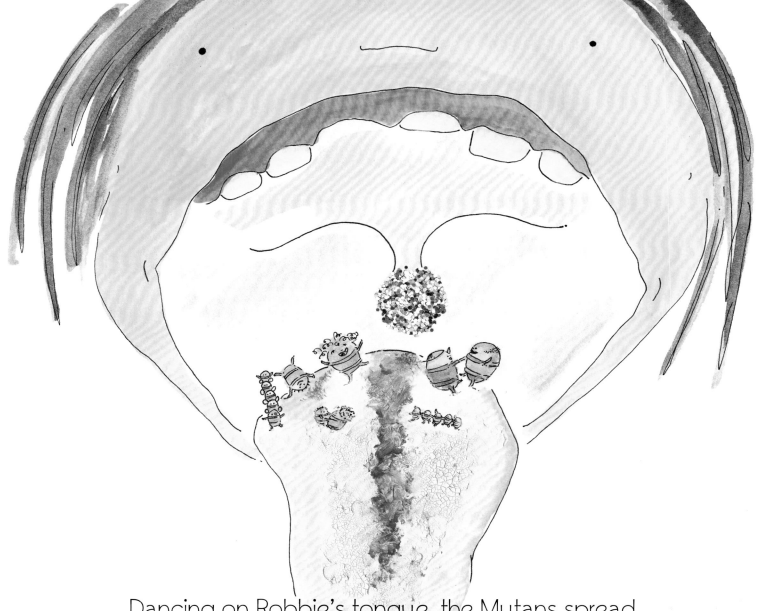

Dancing on Robbie's tongue, the Mutans spread
a thick layer of gunk, making it sticky and slimy.

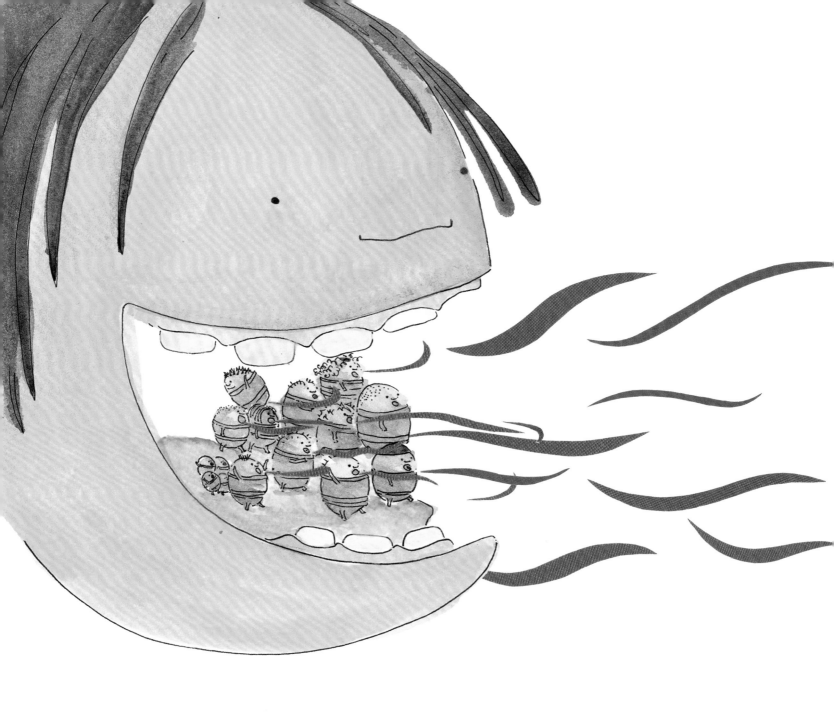

The Mutans kids blew their stinky breath all over Robbie's friends.

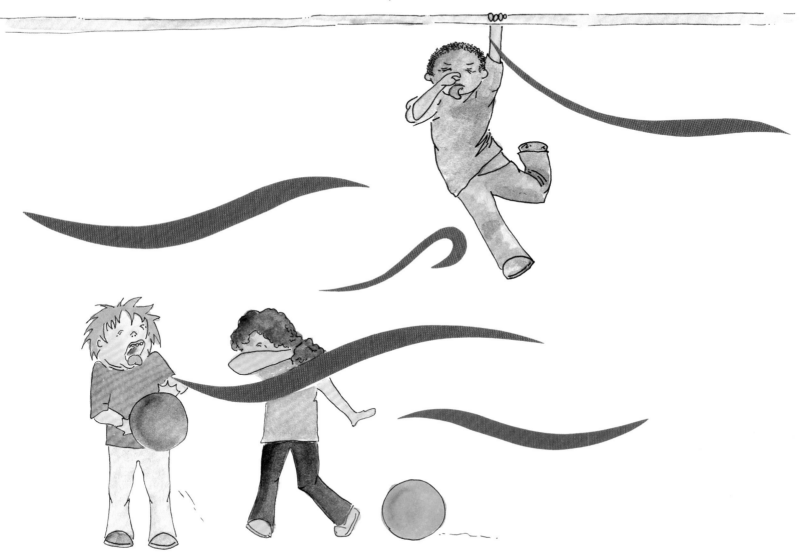

When Robbie painfully chewed his favorite sprinkle donut, his parents finally decided it was time to see the dentist to fix his sugar bug problems.

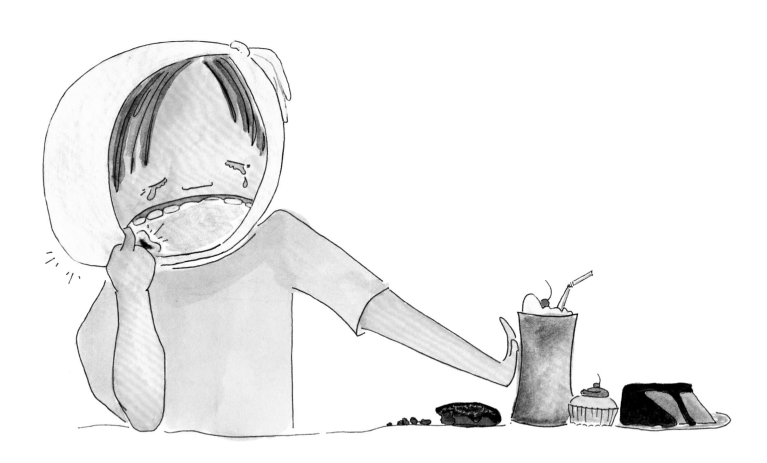

At the dentist's office, Robbie played
in the waiting room.

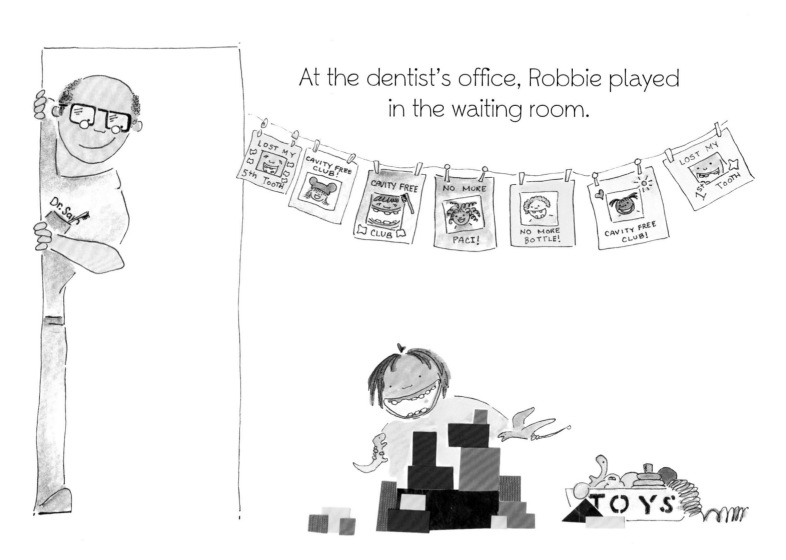

With a big smile, the dentist, Dr. Sam, came out to see Robbie.

Dr. Sam led Robbie to a room with a large comfy chair.
He showed Robbie the amazing instruments used to clean teeth.

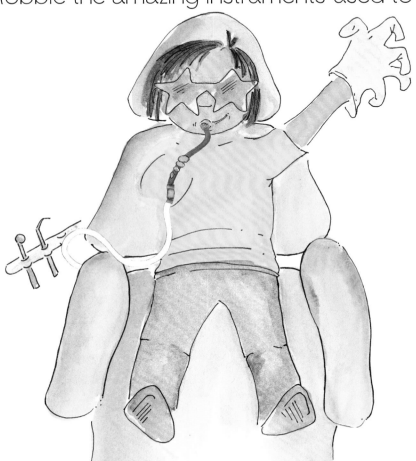

There were sunglasses for Robbie to wear, a water whistler,
a tooth pillow, tooth shampoo, and Mr. Thirsty to hold.

Dr. Sam looked inside Robbie's mouth and found the Mutans' home. He saw the cracks, holes, yellow and brown spots. He felt the bleeding gums. He smelled his sour breath.

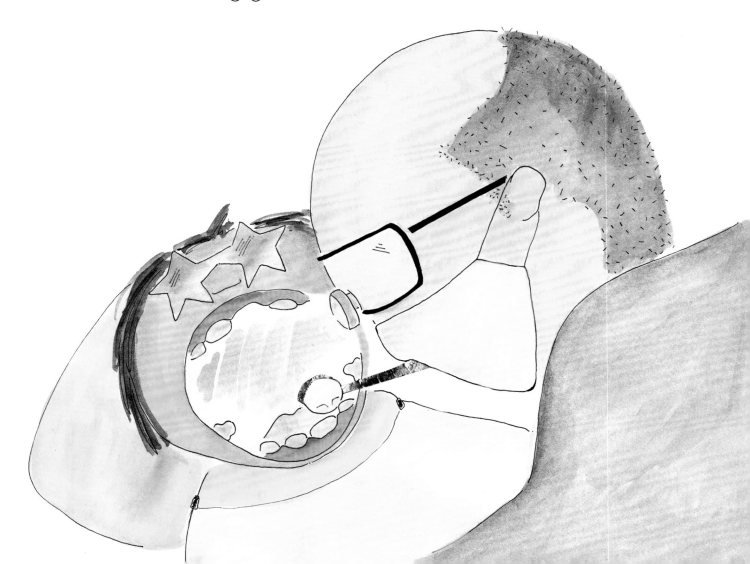

"Robbie, the family of sugar bugs living in your mouth made cavities in your teeth!"

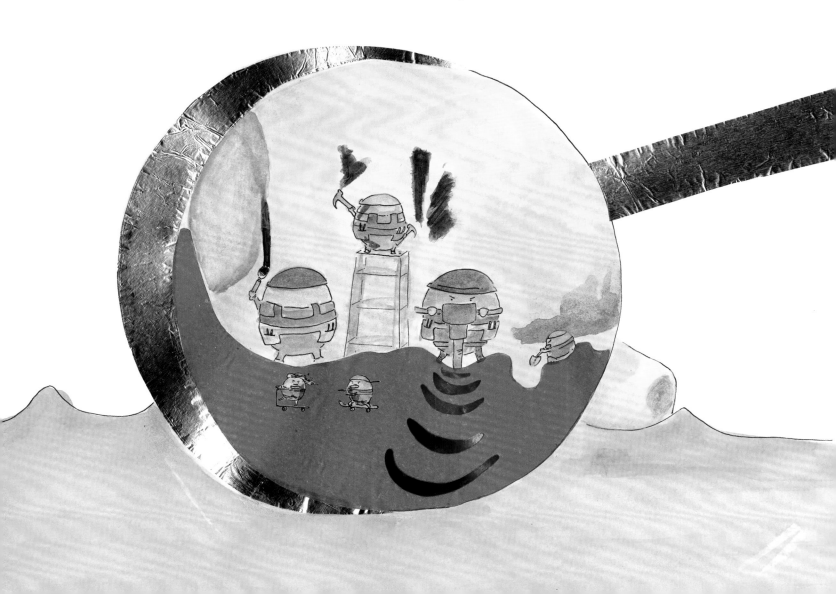

The holes that the Mutans made in Robbie's teeth were fixable.
To stop another family like the Mutans from moving in,
Dr. Sam made Robbie promise to follow three rules:

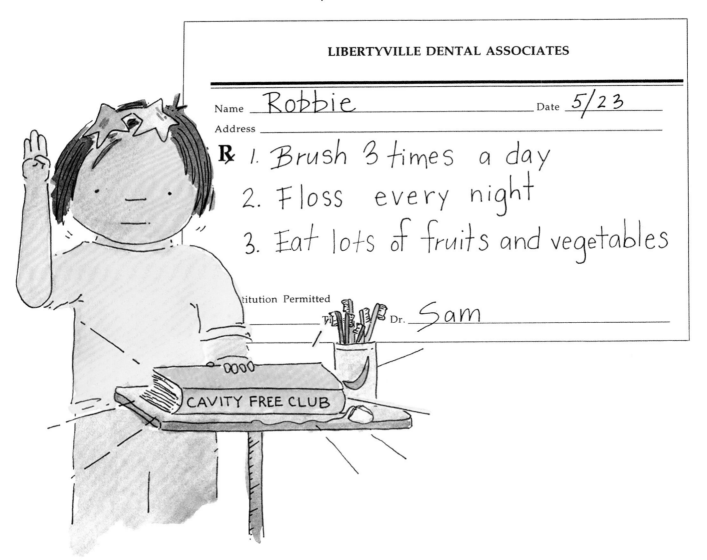

LIBERTYVILLE DENTAL ASSOCIATES

Name __Robbie__   Date __5/23__

Address _____

R 1. Brush 3 times a day

   2. Floss every night

   3. Eat lots of fruits and vegetables

titution Permitted   Dr. __Sam__

CAVITY FREE CLUB

Dr. Sam brushed the whole Mutans family
out of Robbie's mouth through Mr. Thirsty...

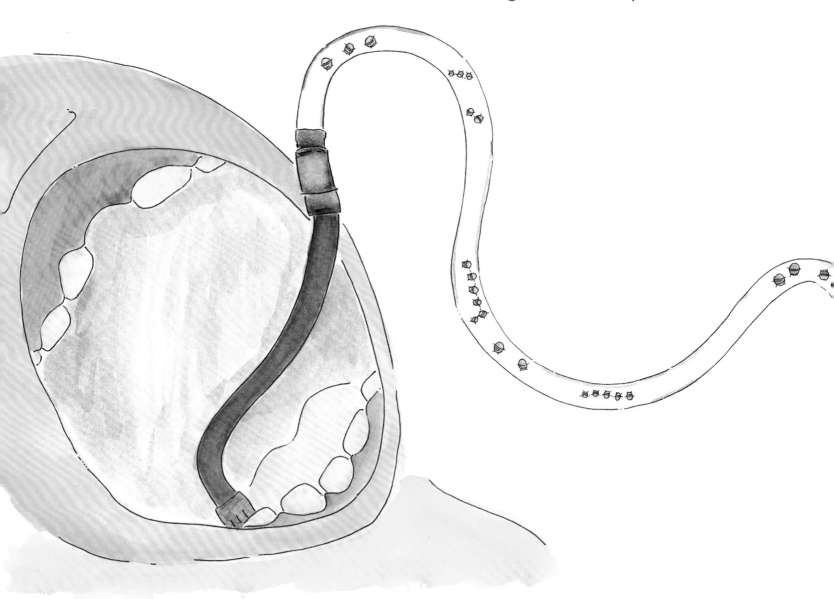

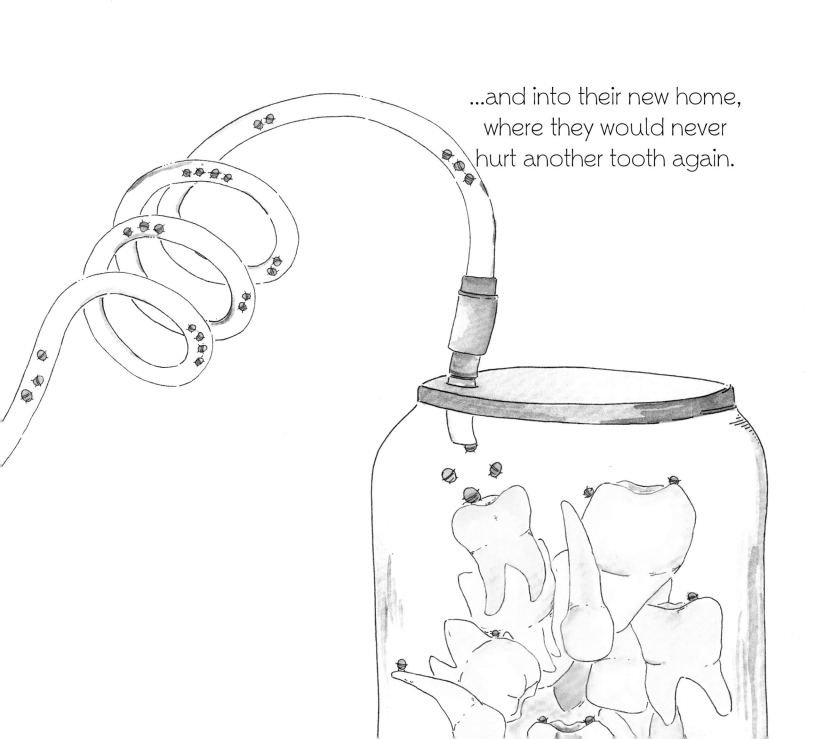

...and into their new home, where they would never hurt another tooth again.

That next morning, Robbie's teeth felt so much better.

But at breakfast Robbie had a choice to make...

As he went to grab his favorite gummies,
he remembered what Dr. Sam taught him.

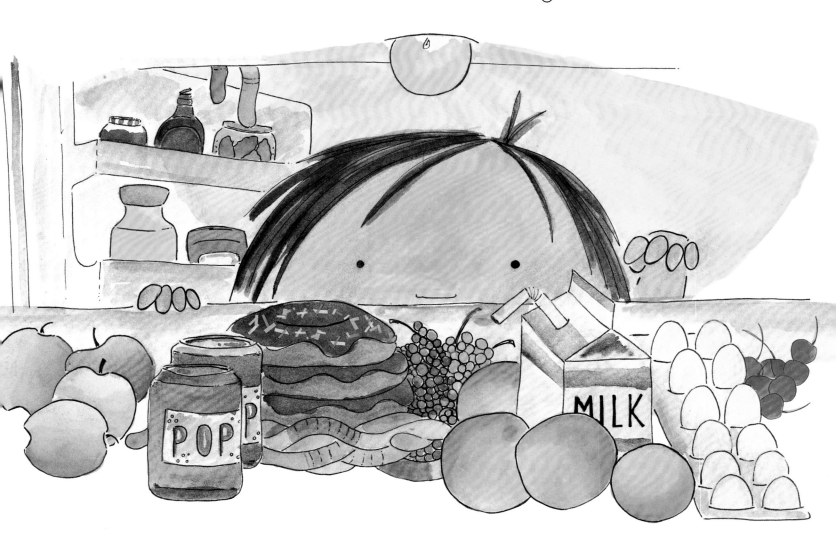

Robbie chose the apple and scrambled eggs
and skipped to school to show off his brand new smile.

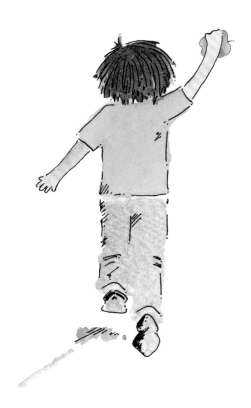

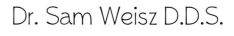The Mutans family was inspired by your own cavity bugs,
streptococcus mutans. They play an important role in causing
cavities by feeding on sugars in your mouth.
With these sugars S. Mutans create acid that leads to
tooth decay and extra visits to the dentist.
With the help of Robbie and the Mutans family, we hope to
inspire your children to stay in the cavity free club
through good home care and fun, easy visits to the dentist.

Dr. Sam Weisz D.D.S.

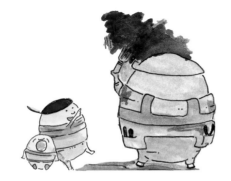

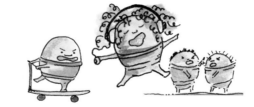

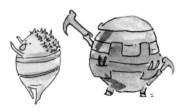

_____ 's 6 Month Check-Up Log

My Dentist: _____   Phone Number: _____

Are Mutans living in *your* mouth?

Date	Oral Hygiene + Home Care	Diet	Number of Cavities	Dentist Initials
	☺ ☐ ☹	☺ ☐ ☹		
	☺ ☐ ☹	☺ ☐ ☹		
	☺ ☐ ☹	☺ ☐ ☹		
	☺ ☐ ☹	☺ ☐ ☹		
	☺ ☐ ☹	☺ ☐ ☹		

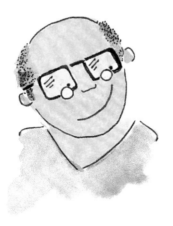

Dr. Sam Weisz D.D.S practices family dentistry
in Libertyville, IL. As a dentist, writer, and dad,
his goal is to inspire a healthy, cavity free lifestyle.
Dr. Sam provides a safe and fun place
for all patients through friendship and humor.
Connect with Dr. Sam Weisz at his office or through
www.askmydentisttv.com

Erica Weisz is a Chicago-born teacher, artist, writer,
and fisherman. Erica's passion for teaching children
inspires her to write and illustrate children's books
that focus on character building, self-discovery,
and personal growth. Connect with Erica Weisz at
www.mrsweiszbooks.com

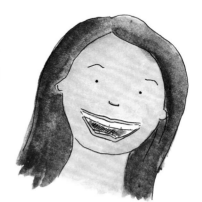